Osteoporosis Exercise for Beginners

Understanding the Importance of Osteoporosis Exercise

By

Alden Keelan

Table of Contents

CHAPTER 1

Introduction

1.1 Understanding Osteoporosis

Osteoporosis is a widespread and potentially debilitating medical condition that affects the skeletal system, leading to fragile and porous bones. To understand osteoporosis, it's crucial to delve into the intricate workings of the human skeletal system and the factors that contribute to this condition.

The Human Skeletal System:

The skeletal system serves as the structural framework of the body, providing support, protection for vital organs, and facilitating movement. It comprises bones, which are living tissues that constantly undergo a process of regeneration and renewal. Bones are primarily composed of collagen, a strong protein, and minerals such as calcium and phosphorus, which give them their hardness and density.

Osteoporosis Defined:

Osteoporosis, which translates to "porous bone," is characterized by a loss of bone density and a deterioration of bone structure. This results in bones becoming fragile and more susceptible to fractures, even from minor stresses like a fall or a bump. It is often referred to as a "silent disease" because it progresses silently, without any noticeable symptoms until a fracture occurs.

Causes of Osteoporosis:

1. **Age:** Osteoporosis is more common in older adults because bone density naturally decreases with age. This process is accelerated in women after menopause due to hormonal changes.

2. **Hormonal Factors:** Hormones play a crucial role in maintaining bone density. Reductions in estrogen (in women) and testosterone (in men) can contribute to bone loss. Conditions like early menopause, low body weight, or hormone-related disorders can increase the risk.

3. **Nutrition and Diet:** Inadequate calcium and vitamin D intake can weaken bones. Additionally, certain medical conditions and

medications can interfere with nutrient absorption or bone metabolism.

4. **Lifestyle Choices:** Sedentary lifestyles, smoking, excessive alcohol consumption, and low physical activity levels can all contribute to the development of osteoporosis.

5. **Genetics:** Family history and genetics can also influence a person's susceptibility to osteoporosis.

1.2 Importance of Exercise

Exercise is an essential component in the management and prevention of osteoporosis. It plays a pivotal role in maintaining bone health and can significantly reduce the risk of fractures associated with this condition. Here's why exercise is crucial:

Strengthening Bones: Weight-bearing exercises, such as walking, jogging, and resistance training, subject bones to stress, which in turn stimulates bone growth and remodeling. This helps to maintain or increase bone density.

Improving Balance and Coordination: Osteoporosis can increase the risk of falls and fractures. Exercises that enhance balance, like yoga or tai chi, can reduce this risk by improving stability and coordination.

Muscle Strength: Strong muscles can provide additional support to the bones, reducing the risk of falls and fractures. Resistance training, using weights or resistance bands, is particularly effective in building muscle strength.

Joint Flexibility: Regular exercise keeps joints flexible and mobile, which can help maintain overall mobility and reduce the risk of falls.

Enhancing Overall Health: Exercise offers a multitude of other health benefits, including cardiovascular health, weight management, and mood improvement. These benefits are particularly important for individuals with osteoporosis, as they can contribute to a better quality of life.

osteoporosis is a condition characterized by weakened and porous bones, making individuals more susceptible to fractures. Understanding the factors that contribute to osteoporosis is essential for its prevention and management. Exercise plays a vital role in this process by strengthening bones, improving balance, and enhancing overall health. It is a cornerstone in the fight against osteoporosis, promoting not only bone health but also a better quality of life for those affected by this condition.

CHAPTER 2

Assessing Your Health

2.1 Medical Evaluation

A comprehensive medical evaluation is a critical initial step in assessing your health when dealing with osteoporosis or potential risk factors for this condition. This evaluation involves a thorough examination by a healthcare provider to understand your overall health, medical history, and risk factors related to osteoporosis.

The Components of a Medical Evaluation for Osteoporosis:

1. **Medical History:** Your healthcare provider will start by gathering information about your personal and family medical history. This includes any previous fractures, medical conditions, medications you are currently taking, and lifestyle factors like smoking and alcohol consumption.

2. **Physical Examination:** A physical examination may be performed to assess your general health and to look for any visible signs of osteoporosis, such as postural changes or height loss.

3. **Fracture Risk Assessment:** Your healthcare provider will use established tools and guidelines to assess your risk of fractures. They may consider factors like age, sex, family history, and medical conditions.

4. **Medication Review:** If you are currently taking medications, especially those known to affect bone health (e.g., corticosteroids), your provider will evaluate their impact on your bone health and discuss potential alternatives or adjustments.

5. **Nutritional Assessment:** A review of your diet and nutritional intake, especially calcium and vitamin D, is important to ensure you are getting the necessary nutrients for bone health.

6. **Lifestyle Factors:** Your healthcare provider will discuss lifestyle factors that can influence bone health, such as physical activity levels, smoking, and alcohol consumption. They may provide guidance on making healthier choices.

7. **Other Medical Conditions:**
    Certain medical conditions, such as hormonal disorders or gastrointestinal issues, can affect nutrient absorption and bone health. These will be considered in the evaluation.

2.2 Bone Density Testing

Bone density testing, also known as bone densitometry or dual-energy x-ray absorptiometry (DEXA), is a specialized diagnostic test used to measure bone mineral density (BMD). It is a critical component of osteoporosis assessment and helps determine the strength and density of your bones.

Key Aspects of Bone Density Testing:

1. **Non-Invasive Procedure:** Bone density testing is a non-invasive and painless procedure. It typically focuses on areas prone to fractures, such as the hip and spine.

2. **Measurement of Bone Density:** The test measures the amount of mineral in your bones, primarily calcium. A T-score is generated, which compares your BMD to that of a healthy young adult of the same sex. A Z-score may also be provided, which compares your BMD to that of people your own age.

3. **Identification of Osteoporosis:** The results of the bone density test can help diagnose osteoporosis, classify its severity (mild, moderate, severe), and assess the risk of future fractures.

4. **Monitoring Progress:** Bone density testing can be used for monitoring changes in bone density over time, which is important for evaluating the effectiveness of treatment or lifestyle changes.

5. **Frequency:** How often you need bone density testing depends on your individual risk factors and the results of previous tests. Generally, it may be recommended every 1 to 2 years for individuals at higher risk.

6. **Risk Assessment Tool:** The World Health Organization's FRAX tool may be used in conjunction with bone density testing to estimate your 10-year risk of experiencing a major osteoporotic fracture.

Assessing your health when dealing with osteoporosis involves a thorough medical evaluation, including a review of medical history, risk factors, medications, and lifestyle. Bone density testing is a key diagnostic tool used to measure bone mineral density and assess your risk of fractures. These assessments are crucial for early detection, diagnosis, and management of osteoporosis, allowing healthcare providers to develop appropriate treatment and prevention plans tailored to your specific needs.

CHAPTER 3

Safety Precautions

3.1 Consultation with a Healthcare Provider

Before embarking on any exercise program, especially if you have osteoporosis or osteoporosis-related risk factors, it is essential to consult with a healthcare provider. This step ensures that your exercise plan is safe and tailored to your specific health needs.

Key Aspects of Consultation with a Healthcare Provider:

1. **Medical History Review:** Your healthcare provider will review your medical history, including

any previous fractures, surgeries, chronic conditions, and medications you are currently taking. This information helps them assess your overall health and any specific concerns related to osteoporosis.

2. **Fracture Risk Assessment:** Your provider will evaluate your risk of fractures based on various factors, including your age, sex, family history, and bone density test results. This assessment guides exercise recommendations.

3. **Medication Evaluation:** If you are taking medications for osteoporosis or other conditions, your healthcare provider will assess their impact on your bone health and discuss any exercise-related precautions or recommendations.

4. **Physical Examination:** A physical examination may be conducted to check for any physical limitations or medical conditions that might affect your exercise plan.

5. **Exercise Prescription:** Based on your medical history and assessment, your healthcare provider may prescribe specific exercises, recommend exercise intensity, and provide guidance on exercise duration and frequency.

6. **Clearance for Exercise:** Your provider will give you clearance to begin or continue with an exercise program, ensuring that it is safe for your individual circumstances.

3.2 Identifying Exercise Limitations

Identifying exercise limitations is crucial to ensure your safety while exercising with osteoporosis. These limitations are often determined through the consultation with your healthcare provider and may include:

1. **Specific Movement Restrictions:** Depending on your bone density and fracture risk, your healthcare provider may advise against certain high-impact activities that could increase the risk of fractures, such as jumping or vigorous running.

2. **Weight-Bearing Considerations:** If you have severe osteoporosis, you may need to avoid activities that place excessive stress on your

spine and hips, such as heavy lifting or high-impact aerobics.

3. **Balance and Coordination Challenges:** If you have difficulty with balance or coordination, you may need to focus on exercises that improve these skills to reduce the risk of falls.

4. **Exercise Modifications:** Some exercises may need to be modified to reduce the risk of injury. For example, using lighter weights or resistance bands for strength training or performing modified yoga poses.

3.3 Creating a Safe Exercise Environment

Creating a safe exercise environment is essential to minimize the risk of accidents and injuries, especially when you have osteoporosis. Here are key considerations:

1. **Supportive Surfaces:** Exercise on surfaces that provide adequate support and cushioning, such as exercise mats or stable floors.

2. **Proper Footwear:** Wear appropriate footwear with good arch support and non-slip soles to reduce the risk of falls.

3. **Clear Space:** Ensure that the exercise area is free of obstacles or hazards that could cause tripping or falling.

4. **Use of Assistive Devices:** If needed, use assistive devices like balance aids or handrails to enhance stability during exercises.

5. **Supervision:** If you are new to exercise or have specific limitations, consider exercising under the supervision of a qualified fitness professional who can provide guidance and ensure proper technique.

6. **Emergency Plan:** Have a plan in place in case of emergencies, including access to a phone and knowledge of what to do if an injury occurs.

safety precautions when exercising with osteoporosis involve consulting with a healthcare provider to assess your individual health status, identifying exercise limitations, and creating a safe exercise environment. These measures are essential for reducing the risk of fractures and

injuries while promoting the benefits
of exercise for bone health and overall
well-being.

CHAPTER 4

Types of Osteoporosis-Friendly Exercises

4.1 Weight-Bearing Exercises

Weight-bearing exercises involve activities that require you to support your body's weight through your bones and muscles. These exercises are particularly beneficial for osteoporosis because they help stimulate bone growth and maintain bone density.

4.1.1 Walking

Walking is one of the most accessible and effective weight-bearing exercises for individuals with osteoporosis. It is a low-impact activity that places minimal stress on the joints while providing excellent bone-strengthening benefits. Aim for at least 30 minutes of brisk walking most days of the week to reap the rewards.

4.1.2 Dancing

Dancing, whether it's ballroom, salsa, or even line dancing, is a fun and social way to engage in weight-bearing exercise. Dancing involves varied movements, including weight shifts and steps, which help improve balance and coordination in addition to promoting bone health.

4.1.3 Stair Climbing

Climbing stairs is another weight-bearing exercise that challenges your leg muscles and bones. If you have access to a staircase, consider incorporating stair climbing into your routine. Start slowly and gradually increase the number of flights of stairs you climb.

4.2 Strength Training

Strength training, also known as resistance training, focuses on building muscle strength. It's essential for individuals with osteoporosis because strong muscles provide additional support to the bones, reducing the risk of falls and fractures.

4.2.1 Resistance Bands

Resistance bands are excellent tools for strength training, especially for beginners with osteoporosis. They provide resistance without the need for heavy weights, reducing the risk of injury. You can perform a variety of exercises with resistance bands to target different muscle groups.

4.2.2 Bodyweight Exercises

Bodyweight exercises use your own body weight as resistance. These exercises include squats, lunges, push-ups, and planks. They can be adapted to your fitness level, making them suitable for individuals of all abilities.

4.2.3 Dumbbell Exercises

Dumbbell exercises involve lifting weights to build muscle strength. For individuals with osteoporosis, it's important to start with light weights and proper form to avoid injury. Common dumbbell exercises include bicep curls, tricep extensions, and chest presses.

Additional Considerations:

1. **Proper Form:** Regardless of the type of exercise you choose, proper form is crucial. Incorrect form can lead to injuries. If you're new to these exercises, consider working with a qualified fitness trainer to ensure you're using correct form.

2. **Progression:** Start slowly and gradually increase the intensity and duration of your exercises over time. This gradual progression is essential for building strength and reducing the risk of injury.

3. **Rest and Recovery:** Allow your body sufficient time to rest and recover between exercise sessions. Adequate rest is when your body repairs and strengthens itself.

4. **Consult Your Healthcare Provider:** Before starting any new exercise program, especially if you have osteoporosis, consult with your healthcare provider or a physical therapist. They can provide guidance and ensure that your exercise plan is safe and appropriate for your specific condition.

Incorporating a combination of weight-bearing exercises and strength training into your routine can help improve bone health, muscle strength, and overall physical well-being for individuals with osteoporosis.

4.3 Flexibility and Balance Exercises

Flexibility and balance exercises are essential components of an osteoporosis-friendly exercise routine. These exercises help improve your range of motion, enhance posture, and reduce the risk of falls and fractures.

4.3.1 Yoga

Yoga is a mind-body practice that combines physical postures, controlled breathing, and meditation. It's particularly beneficial for individuals with osteoporosis for several reasons:

- **Improved Flexibility:** Yoga involves a variety of stretches and poses that can enhance flexibility and joint mobility.

- **Balance Enhancement:** Many yoga poses require balance and stability, which can help reduce the risk of falls.

- **Stress Reduction:** Yoga promotes relaxation and stress reduction, which can benefit both physical and mental well-being.

When practicing yoga with osteoporosis, it's important to choose classes or instructors who are knowledgeable about modifications for osteoporosis and can guide you in using proper alignment to prevent injury.

4.3.2 Tai Chi

Tai Chi is a low-impact, slow-moving martial art that focuses on balance, coordination, and flexibility. It's particularly beneficial for individuals with osteoporosis because:

- **Improved Balance:** Tai Chi emphasizes weight shifting and controlled movements, which enhance balance and reduce the risk of falls.

- **Joint Flexibility:** The gentle, flowing movements of Tai Chi can improve joint flexibility and reduce stiffness.

- **Stress Reduction:** Similar to yoga, Tai Chi promotes relaxation and mental well-being.

Tai Chi classes are widely available and are often suitable for people of all fitness levels. It can be a enjoyable and social way to improve balance and flexibility.

4.3.3 Balance Exercises

Balance exercises specifically target your stability and coordination. They can be incorporated into your daily routine and are essential for fall prevention. Here are some balance exercises you can try:

- **Single-leg balance:** Stand on one leg and hold the position for as long as you can. Repeat on the other leg. You can use a chair or wall for support if needed.

- **Heel-to-toe walk:** Walk in a straight line, placing one foot directly in front of the other, heel to toe. This mimics a sobriety test and challenges your balance.

- **Balance on one foot while closing your eyes:** This exercise increases the difficulty by removing visual cues, forcing your body to rely solely on proprioception (awareness of body position).

- **Standing leg lifts:** Lift one leg to the side while maintaining balance on the other. Hold for a few seconds, then switch to the other leg.

- **Balancing on a cushion:** Stand on a cushion or foam pad to make your balance exercises more challenging.

Balance exercises can be practiced daily and can be easily integrated into your daily routine, such as while brushing your teeth or waiting in line.

Incorporating flexibility and balance exercises like yoga, Tai Chi, and balance-specific routines into your osteoporosis-friendly exercise plan not only enhances your physical capabilities but also reduces the risk of falls, which can be particularly concerning for individuals with fragile bones. Always start slowly, progress gradually, and consult with a healthcare provider or physical therapist if you have any concerns about your balance or mobility.

CHAPTER 5

Developing a Custom Exercise Plan

Creating a custom exercise plan for osteoporosis involves careful consideration of your individual needs, abilities, and goals. Here are essential steps to guide you through this process:

5.1 Setting Realistic Goals

Setting realistic and achievable goals is a crucial first step in developing an effective exercise plan for osteoporosis. Your goals should align with your current fitness level and take into account any limitations or health concerns. Here's how to set goals effectively:

1. **Consult Your Healthcare Provider:** Discuss your exercise goals with your healthcare provider to ensure they are safe and appropriate for your specific health condition and any medications you may be taking.

2. **Identify Your Objectives:** Determine what you want to achieve through exercise. Are your goals focused on improving bone density, building muscle strength, enhancing balance, reducing pain, or a combination of these factors?

3. **Be Specific:** Set specific and measurable goals. For example,

rather than saying "I want to improve my bone health," specify "I want to increase my bone density by X% in Y months."

4. **Consider Short-Term and Long-Term Goals:** Break down your goals into short-term and long-term objectives. Short-term goals help you stay motivated and track progress, while long-term goals provide a broader perspective.

5. **Realistic Expectations:** Be realistic about what you can achieve within a given timeframe. Understand that progress may be gradual, especially if you're new to exercise.

6. **Flexibility:** Allow for flexibility in your goals to adapt to any changes in your health or circumstances.

5.2 Frequency and Duration

The frequency and duration of your exercise plan will depend on your goals, current fitness level, and the type of exercises you choose. Here are some general guidelines:

1. **Frequency:** How often you exercise each week will vary based on your goals and the intensity of your workouts. A common recommendation is to aim for at least 150 minutes of moderate-intensity aerobic activity or 75 minutes of vigorous-intensity aerobic activity per week, spread throughout the week. This can be divided into sessions of 30 minutes, five days a week.

2. **Aerobic Exercise:** For aerobic exercises like walking, dancing, or

stair climbing, aim for at least 3-5 sessions per week. Start with shorter sessions and gradually increase the duration as your fitness level improves.

3. **Strength Training:** Strength training exercises should target major muscle groups and be performed at least 2-3 times a week. Allow a day of rest between strength training sessions to give your muscles time to recover.

4. **Flexibility and Balance:** Incorporate flexibility and balance exercises like yoga or Tai Chi into your routine 2-3 times a week. These can be performed daily for shorter durations.

5. **Progression:** As you become more comfortable with your exercise routine, gradually

increase the duration, intensity, or complexity of your workouts. Progression is essential for continued improvement.

6. **Rest and Recovery:** Don't forget to include rest days in your exercise plan. Your body needs time to recover and repair itself.

7. **Listen to Your Body:** Pay attention to how your body responds to exercise. If you experience pain, discomfort, or unusual fatigue, consult your healthcare provider or a qualified fitness professional.

your exercise plan should be adaptable to your changing needs and progress. Regularly review your goals and modify your plan accordingly to ensure that it remains effective and motivating. It's also important to track your progress and celebrate your achievements along the way to stay motivated and focused on your long-term health goals.

5.3 Progression and Variation

Progression and variation are key principles in developing a successful and sustainable exercise plan, especially when dealing with osteoporosis. These principles ensure that your workouts remain effective, engaging, and safe over time. Here's how to incorporate progression and variation into your exercise routine:

Progression:

1. **Gradual Intensity Increase:** As your fitness level improves, gradually increase the intensity of

your exercises. For aerobic activities like walking, consider walking faster or tackling more challenging terrain. In strength training, slowly increase the weight or resistance you use.

2. **Additional Sets and Repetitions:** In strength training, as you become more comfortable with a particular exercise, add more sets and repetitions to continue challenging your muscles.

3. **Advanced Variations:** As your skills improve, you can introduce more advanced variations of exercises. For example, in yoga, you might progress from basic poses to more challenging ones.

4. **Regular Reassessment:** Periodically reassess your goals and fitness level. Adjust your

exercise plan to match your current capabilities and objectives. This may involve consulting with a fitness professional or your healthcare provider.

5. **Cross-Training:** Incorporate different types of exercises into your routine to work different muscle groups and avoid overuse injuries. For example, mix strength training with aerobic exercises like swimming or cycling.

6. **Tracking Progress:** Keep a record of your workouts, noting the number of sets, repetitions, weights, or durations. Tracking your progress can help you see improvements and identify areas that may need more attention.

Variation:

1. **Exercise Selection:** Include a variety of exercises in your routine to prevent boredom and engage different muscle groups. For example, if you typically walk for cardio, consider mixing in swimming or dancing for variety.

2. **Change Workout Environment:** Sometimes, simply changing where you exercise can add excitement. Take your workout outdoors or to a new gym or fitness class.

3. **Different Modalities:** Explore different exercise modalities. In addition to traditional weightlifting, try bodyweight exercises, resistance bands, or exercise machines. In yoga, experiment with different styles and classes.

4. **Group Activities:** Join group exercise classes or activities. Group settings can be motivating and introduce you to new exercises or routines.

5. **Interval Training:** Incorporate interval training into your aerobic workouts. This involves alternating between periods of higher intensity and lower intensity, which can boost cardiovascular fitness and prevent exercise plateaus.

6. **Periodization:** Consider a periodization approach, which involves breaking your training into distinct cycles with varying goals and intensities. This can help prevent burnout and enhance long-term progress.

7. **Mind-Body Practices:** Include mind-body practices like meditation or deep breathing exercises as part of your routine. These practices can help reduce stress and improve overall well-being.

Incorporating both progression and variation into your exercise plan, you can ensure that your workouts remain effective, engaging, and safe. Remember that your exercise plan should be enjoyable and sustainable over the long term. If you ever have concerns or questions about your exercise routine, don't hesitate to consult with a qualified fitness professional or healthcare provider for guidance and adjustments.

CHAPTER 6

Proper Technique and Form

Maintaining proper technique and form during exercise is essential for preventing injuries, optimizing results, and ensuring that your osteoporosis-friendly exercise routine is safe and effective. Here are key aspects of proper technique and form:

6.1 Warm-Up and Cool-Down

6.1.1 Warm-Up

A proper warm-up prepares your body for exercise by increasing blood flow to your muscles and gradually

elevating your heart rate. This helps
reduce the risk of injury and prepares
your body for more intense activity. A
warm-up should include:

- **Aerobic Activity:** Start with 5-10
  minutes of low-intensity aerobic
  activity, such as brisk walking or
  gentle cycling.

- **Dynamic Stretching:** Include
  dynamic stretches that mimic the
  movements you'll be doing during
  your workout. For example, leg
  swings or arm circles can be
  effective.

6.1.2 Cool-Down

After your workout, a cool-down
helps your body return to its pre-
exercise state, gradually lowering
your heart rate and reducing the risk
of muscle soreness. A cool-down
should include:

- **Static Stretching:** Perform static stretches that target the muscles you worked during your exercise. Hold each stretch for 15-30 seconds without bouncing.

- **Deep Breathing:** Incorporate deep breathing exercises to relax and calm your body.

6.2 Breathing Techniques

Proper breathing is crucial for maintaining oxygen supply to your muscles, regulating blood pressure, and preventing fatigue during exercise. Here are some breathing techniques to consider:

- **Aerobic Exercise:** During aerobic activities like walking or dancing, maintain a steady and rhythmic breathing pattern. Inhale through your nose and exhale through your mouth. The rate of breathing should match the intensity of your exercise.

- **Strength Training:** When lifting weights or performing resistance exercises, exhale during the effort phase (e.g., lifting the weight) and inhale during the relaxation phase. Avoid holding your breath, as it can increase blood pressure and strain.

- **Yoga and Tai Chi:** In these mind-body practices, breathing is often coordinated with specific movements. Follow the breathing instructions provided by your instructor, which can vary depending on the style and pose.

- **Awareness:** Pay attention to your breathing throughout your workout. It can help you stay focused and maintain proper form.

6.3 Posture and Alignment

Maintaining proper posture and alignment is crucial for preventing injuries, optimizing the effectiveness of your exercises, and reducing strain on your bones and joints. Here are some guidelines for maintaining good posture and alignment:

- **Head and Neck:** Keep your head in a neutral position, looking straight ahead. Avoid tilting your head up or down excessively.

- **Shoulders:** Relax your shoulders and keep them down and back, not hunched forward.

- **Spine:** Maintain a straight and neutral spine when performing exercises. Avoid excessive arching or rounding of the back.

- **Core Engagement:** Engage your core muscles to support your spine and maintain stability. This is particularly important during strength training exercises.

- **Hips:** Keep your hips level and aligned with your spine. Avoid excessive tilting or twisting of the hips.

- **Knees and Ankles:** Align your knees and ankles with your hips and feet. Avoid inward or outward rotation of the knees.

- **Feet:** Maintain a stable base of support with your feet. In weight-bearing exercises, distribute your weight evenly between both feet.

- **Mirrors or Feedback:** Use mirrors or ask a workout partner or instructor for feedback on your form and posture.

Proper technique and form may vary depending on the type of exercise you're performing. If you're new to a particular exercise or have concerns about your form, consider working with a qualified fitness professional or instructor who can provide guidance and corrections to ensure that you perform exercises safely and effectively.

CHAPTER 7
Tips for Staying Motivated

Staying motivated to exercise regularly, especially when dealing with a health condition like osteoporosis, can be challenging. Here are some tips to help you stay on track:

7.1 Finding a Workout Buddy

Exercising with a partner or workout buddy can make your fitness journey more enjoyable and motivate you to stay consistent. Here's how:

- **Accountability:** Having a workout buddy holds you accountable. You're less likely to skip workouts when someone is relying on you to be there.

- **Friendly Competition:** A little healthy competition can be motivating. Challenge your workout partner to push their limits, and they'll do the same for you.

- **Social Connection:** Exercising with a friend or family member provides an opportunity for social interaction, making your workouts feel like a fun and social activity rather than a chore.

- **Support System:** Your workout buddy can provide emotional support during challenging times and celebrate your successes with you.

7.2 Tracking Your Progress

Monitoring your progress can be a powerful motivator. Here's how to do it effectively:

- **Keep a Workout Journal:** Record your workouts, including the type, duration, and intensity of exercises. Note any milestones or improvements you achieve.

- **Use Fitness Apps:** There are many fitness apps available that can help you track your workouts, set goals, and visualize your progress.

- **Take Photos:** Periodically take photos of yourself. Visual evidence of your changing physique can be incredibly motivating.

- **Measurements:** Track physical measurements like weight, body fat percentage, and waist circumference. These can provide concrete evidence of your progress.

- **Set Achievable Goals:** Establish both short-term and long-term goals. As you achieve these goals, set new ones to keep yourself challenged.

- **Celebrate Milestones:** Celebrate your achievements, no matter how small. Recognizing your successes can boost motivation.

7.3 Incorporating Enjoyable Activities

Exercise doesn't have to be a chore. Find activities you genuinely enjoy to make your workouts something to look forward to:

- **Explore Different Activities:** Try a variety of exercises until you find what you enjoy the most. It could be anything from dancing to hiking, swimming to yoga.

- **Make It Social:** Join group fitness classes or sports leagues that align with your interests. The social aspect can make exercise more enjoyable.

- **Play Music or Podcasts:** Listening to your favorite music or engaging podcasts can make your workouts more entertaining.

- **Change Your Scenery:** If possible, exercise in different environments. Take your workouts outdoors, to a park, or a new gym to keep things fresh.

- **Reward Yourself:** Treat yourself to a small reward after completing a challenging workout or reaching a fitness milestone.

- **Create a Fun Routine:** Design a workout routine that includes activities you genuinely look forward to. If you enjoy it, you're more likely to stick with it.

- **Buddy Up:** As mentioned earlier, exercising with a friend can make workouts more enjoyable through companionship and shared motivation.

motivation can ebb and flow. On days when you're not feeling particularly motivated, remind yourself of your goals, the progress you've made, and the benefits of exercise for your overall health and well-being. Building a consistent exercise habit takes time, but with these strategies, you can stay motivated and make exercise a regular part of your life.

CHAPTER 8

Nutrition for Bone Health

Proper nutrition plays a crucial role in maintaining and improving bone health, especially for individuals with osteoporosis. Here are key dietary considerations for bone health:

8.1 Calcium-Rich Foods

Calcium is a vital mineral for bone health because it contributes to bone density and strength. Here are some calcium-rich foods to include in your diet:

- **Dairy Products:** Milk, yogurt, and cheese are excellent sources of calcium. Opt for low-fat or non-fat versions to limit saturated fat intake.

- **Leafy Greens:** Vegetables like kale, collard greens, turnip greens, and bok choy are rich in calcium.

- **Fortified Foods:** Many foods, such as fortified plant-based milk (e.g., almond, soy, rice milk), cereals, and orange juice, contain added calcium.

- **Sardines and Canned Salmon:** These fish are high in calcium, including the soft bones, which are edible.

- **Tofu and Tempeh:** Soy products like tofu and tempeh are calcium-rich and can be used in various dishes.

- **Nuts and Seeds:** Almonds, chia seeds, and sesame seeds are good sources of calcium.

- **Beans and Lentils:** These legumes provide a moderate amount of calcium.

- **Figs:** Dried figs are relatively high in calcium compared to other fruits.

Ensure that you're getting the recommended daily intake of calcium, which varies depending on age and gender but generally ranges from 1,000 to 1,300 milligrams for adults.

8.2 Vitamin D Sources

Vitamin D is essential for calcium absorption and bone health. It helps your body utilize the calcium you

consume. Sources of vitamin D
include:

- **Sunlight:** Your skin can produce
  vitamin D when exposed to direct
  sunlight. Spending about 10-15
  minutes in the sun a few times a
  week can help. However, this may
  vary depending on factors like
  your location and skin tone.

- **Fatty Fish:** Salmon, mackerel, and
  trout are good dietary sources of
  vitamin D.

- **Fortified Foods:** Many foods,
  including dairy products, plant-
  based milk, cereals, and orange
  juice, are fortified with vitamin D.

- **Supplements:** If you have limited
  sun exposure or difficulty
  obtaining enough vitamin D
  through food, your healthcare

provider may recommend supplements.

Ensure that you meet your daily vitamin D requirements, which typically range from 600 to 800 International Units (IU) for adults.

8.3 Other Nutrients for Bone Health

In addition to calcium and vitamin D, other nutrients contribute to bone health:

- **Magnesium:** This mineral is essential for calcium absorption and bone development. Magnesium-rich foods include leafy greens, nuts, seeds, whole grains, and legumes.

- **Vitamin K:** Vitamin K plays a role in bone mineralization and helps maintain bone density. Leafy greens (such as kale and spinach), broccoli, and Brussels sprouts are good sources.

- **Protein:** Adequate protein intake is necessary for building and repairing bone tissue. Include lean sources of protein like poultry, fish, beans, and tofu in your diet.

- **Phosphorus:** Phosphorus is another mineral involved in bone health. It is abundant in dairy products, meat, and whole grains.

- **Omega-3 Fatty Acids:** Omega-3s may help reduce inflammation and support bone health. Fatty fish like salmon and walnuts are rich sources.

- **Antioxidants:** Antioxidant-rich foods like berries and fruits can help reduce inflammation and support overall health.

- **Limit Sodium and Caffcine:** Excessive sodium and caffeine intake can lead to calcium loss from bones. Limit high-sodium processed foods and moderate caffeine consumption.

A well-balanced diet that includes a variety of nutrient-rich foods can provide the essential vitamins and minerals necessary for maintaining strong and healthy bones. If you have specific dietary concerns or restrictions, consider consulting a registered dietitian or nutritionist for personalized guidance on optimizing your bone health through nutrition.

CHAPTER 9

Lifestyle Changes for Better Bone Health

9.1 Smoking and Alcohol Cessation

The Impact of Smoking on Bone Health

Smoking is known to have detrimental effects on bone health. It can lead to reduced bone density and increase the risk of fractures. The chemicals in tobacco smoke can interfere with the absorption of calcium, a key mineral for bone strength. Additionally, smoking affects hormonal balance, leading to decreased levels of estrogen in women and testosterone in men, which are important for bone health. If you're a smoker, quitting is one of the best steps you can take for your bone health.

Tips for Quitting Smoking

1. **Seek Support**: Reach out to healthcare professionals or support groups that specialize in smoking cessation. They can provide guidance, resources, and strategies to help you quit.

2. **Set a Quit Date**: Choose a specific date to quit smoking. This can serve as a goal and a starting point for your smoke-free journey.

3. **Identify Triggers**: Recognize situations, emotions, or activities that trigger your smoking habit. Finding healthy alternatives to

cope with these triggers can aid in quitting.

4. **Nicotine Replacement Therapy (NRT)**: NRT, such as nicotine patches or gum, can help manage nicotine withdrawal symptoms as you gradually reduce your nicotine intake.

5. **Lifestyle Changes**: Replace smoking with positive activities like exercise, hobbies, or spending time with supportive friends and family.

The Impact of Alcohol on Bone Health

Excessive alcohol consumption can also have negative effects on bone health. It interferes with the body's ability to absorb calcium and other essential nutrients needed for maintaining strong bones. Moreover, alcohol can affect balance and coordination, increasing the risk of falls and fractures.

Tips for Reducing Alcohol Consumption

1. **Set Limits**: Establish clear limits on how much alcohol you'll consume in a given period. Stick to these limits and avoid binge drinking.

2. **Alternate Choices**: opt for non-alcoholic beverages during social gatherings or when you'd normally have a drink. This can help reduce overall alcohol consumption.

3. **Stay Hydrated**: Drinking plenty of water can help you avoid excessive alcohol intake.

4. **Mindful Drinking**: Pay attention to how much you're consuming and how it makes you feel. This awareness can help you make healthier choices.

5. **Seek Support**: If you find it challenging to cut back on alcohol, consider seeking support from healthcare professionals or support groups that focus on alcohol reduction.

The Benefits of Quitting Smoking and Reducing Alcohol Intake

Making the commitment to quit smoking and reduce alcohol consumption can bring significant benefits to your bone health:

- **Improved Bone Density**: Without the negative effects of smoking and excessive alcohol, your bones can better absorb essential nutrients and minerals.

- **Reduced Fracture Risk**: Stronger bones mean a lower risk of fractures, especially in individuals with osteoporosis.

- **Enhanced Overall Health**: Quitting smoking and moderating alcohol consumption contribute to better cardiovascular health and a decreased risk of chronic diseases.

By taking these steps to improve your lifestyle, you're making a positive impact on your bone health and overall well-being.

9.2 Fall Prevention Strategies

Falls can have serious consequences for individuals with osteoporosis due to the increased risk of fractures. Taking proactive steps to prevent falls is essential for safeguarding your bone health and overall well-being. Here are some effective fall prevention strategies to consider:

Maintain Strong Bones and Muscles

1. **Exercise Regularly**: Engaging in weight-bearing exercises, strength training, and balance-enhancing activities can help improve muscle strength and coordination, reducing the risk of falls.

2. **Get Enough Vitamin D and Calcium**: Adequate intake of vitamin D and calcium supports bone health and strength, contributing to better overall stability.

Create a Safe Environment

3. **Remove Clutter**: Clear walkways in your home by removing obstacles like rugs, cords, and clutter that can increase the risk of tripping.

4. **Secure Handrails and Grab Bars**: Install handrails on staircases and in bathrooms to provide additional support and stability.

5. **Good Lighting**: Ensure all areas of your home are well-lit to help you see potential hazards and navigate safely.

Improve Balance and Coordination

6. **Practice Balance Exercises**: Incorporate balance-enhancing exercises, such as standing on one leg or practicing yoga or tai chi, to improve your overall balance and coordination.

7. **Footwear Matters**: Choose footwear with sturdy, non-slip soles that provide proper support and stability.

Be Mindful of Medications

8. **Review Medications**: Some medications can cause dizziness or affect balance. Consult your healthcare provider to review your medication list and address any concerns.

9. **Use Caution with Sedatives**: Be cautious with medications

that can make you drowsy or affect your alertness. Discuss alternatives with your doctor if needed.

Enhance Home Safety

10. **Install Handrails**: Install handrails in hallways and staircases to provide support when moving around your home.

11. **Secure Bathrooms**: Place non-slip mats in the shower and bathtub, and consider using a shower chair if necessary.

12. **Bedroom Precautions**: Ensure your bedroom is well-lit, and keep a phone and flashlight within reach in case you need assistance during the night.

Regular Check-Ups

13. **Eye Exams**: Regular eye exams help ensure your vision is optimal, reducing the risk of falls due to visual impairment.

14. **Hearing Tests**: Addressing hearing issues can help you remain aware of your surroundings and potential hazards.

Emergency Response Plan

15. **Emergency Contact**: Keep a list of emergency contacts on hand and readily accessible.

16. **Alert System**: Consider using a personal alert system that allows you to call for help in case of a fall or other emergency.

Stay Active and Engaged

17. **Stay Active Socially**: Engaging in social activities helps maintain cognitive function and keeps you connected with a support network.

18. **Mindful Movement**: Be aware of your surroundings and move at a pace that allows you to maintain balance.

Taking these fall prevention strategies seriously can significantly reduce your risk of falls and fractures, promoting both bone health and overall quality of life.

CHAPTER 10

Dealing with Pain and Discomfort

Engaging in exercises can sometimes lead to discomfort or pain, particularly for individuals with osteoporosis. It's important to understand how to recognize pain signals, when to seek medical attention, and how to modify exercises for comfort.

10.1 Recognizing Pain Signals

1. **Differentiating Between Discomfort and Pain**: Discomfort during exercise is common, especially when you're challenging your body. However, sharp or shooting pain is not normal and could indicate an issue.

2. **Localized vs. Radiating Pain**: Pay attention to whether the pain is localized to a specific area or if it's radiating through a larger region. Radiating pain might indicate nerve involvement and should be taken seriously.

3. **Persistent Pain**: If you experience pain that doesn't subside after stopping the exercise or persists for an extended period, it's a sign to pause and evaluate.

10.2 When to Seek Medical Attention

1. **Severe Pain**: If you're experiencing severe pain that limits your movement or is intolerable, stop the exercise immediately and consult a healthcare professional.

2. **Sudden Changes**: If you notice sudden changes in pain intensity, location, or type during an exercise, it's a red flag to stop and seek medical advice.

3. **Unusual Symptoms**: Any symptoms such as numbness, tingling, weakness, or loss of sensation warrant immediate medical attention.

10.3 Modifying Exercises for Comfort

1. **Reducing Impact**: If weight-bearing exercises cause discomfort, consider low-impact alternatives like swimming or stationary cycling.

2. **Range of Motion**: opt for exercises that allow you to stay within a pain-free range of motion. Avoid overstretching or pushing yourself too hard.

3. **Gentle Stretching**: Incorporate gentle stretching after your workout to improve flexibility and alleviate muscle tension.

4. **Proper Technique**: Ensure you're using proper form during exercises. Poor technique can lead

to unnecessary strain and
discomfort.

5. **Consultation with a Professional**:
   If you're unsure about modifying
   exercises, consult a physical
   therapist or fitness professional.
   They can provide guidance
   tailored to your condition.

The goal is to engage in exercises that
challenge you without causing undue
pain or discomfort. It's always better
to be cautious and prioritize your
safety and well-being.

CHAPTER 11

Osteoporosis Medications and Exercise

11.1 Understanding Medication Effects

Managing osteoporosis often involves a combination of medications and lifestyle changes. It's essential to understand how your medications may interact with exercise and impact your bone health:

1. **Bisphosphonates**: These medications slow down bone loss and are commonly prescribed. While rare, some individuals might

experience bone, joint, or muscle pain. If you experience any discomfort during exercise, consult your healthcare provider.

2. **Calcitonin**: This hormone can help manage bone loss and reduce pain associated with fractures. It's important to note that calcitonin is often used alongside other medications. Exercise can complement the effects of calcitonin by promoting bone health and reducing fracture risk.

3. **Hormone Replacement Therapy (HRT)**: HRT, particularly estrogen therapy, can help manage bone loss in postmenopausal women. Exercise can further support bone health by increasing bone density and strength.

4. **Selective Estrogen Receptor Modulators (SERMs)**: These medications mimic the effects of estrogen on bone density. Like HRT, exercise can enhance the benefits of SERMs by promoting bone strength.

5. **Denosumab**: This medication is an alternative for those who can't tolerate bisphosphonates. It's important to note that while it reduces bone resorption, it might slightly increase the risk of rare fractures. Exercise can contribute to overall bone health.

11.2 Communicating with Your Healthcare Provider

1. **Open Dialogue**: When starting a new exercise regimen, inform your healthcare provider about your plans. They can provide insights on how exercises might interact with your medications.

2. **Medication Timing**: Some medications require specific timing, like taking them on an empty stomach. Discuss the best times to exercise to avoid interference with medication absorption.

3. **Symptom Reporting**: If you experience any unusual symptoms or changes while exercising, report them to your healthcare provider. They can determine if the

symptoms are related to your medications or exercise routine.

4. **Adaptations**: Work with your healthcare provider to adapt your exercise routine if needed. Certain medications might require modifications to exercise intensity or types of activities.

5. **Regular Check-Ups**: Attend regular check-ups with your healthcare provider to monitor the effectiveness of both your medications and exercise routine.

Your healthcare provider is your best resource for understanding how osteoporosis medications and exercise interact in your specific case. Their guidance will ensure you're making informed decisions to support your bone health.